THE
CONCISE NUTRITION
AND LIFESTYLE GUIDE

A Practical Plan for Better Health

Dr Philip Bosanquet & Dr Helen Bosanquet

THE CONCISE NUTRITION AND LIFESTYLE GUIDE

CONTENTS

INTRODUCTION

Many changes in the way we live have taken place in the last seventy years. Advances in healthcare and technology can at first glance seem like a long list of successes. Surgery could change that broken bone from what would have been a permanent disability into a short term inconvenience. Easy access to food, transportation, computers and the internet have made certain aspects of life much more convenient.

During this period of change, a huge rise in obesity and chronic health conditions, both physical and mental, has also occurred. This is increasingly affecting children as well as adults. New terms such as 'childhood obesity' have had to be coined. In an ironic twist, it is many of those changes made during the last seventy years, designed to make life better, that have driven the current health crisis. In addition to this, despite more material wealth than at any other time in history, many people in the western world are unhappy.

As doctors working in the NHS, we have repeatedly seen the failure of modern medicine to tackle the root causes of obesity and poor health. As a consequence, much of society is embracing a dangerous delusion that as life goes on, weight gain and disease are inevitable. For many people, the determination to combat this pattern is waning. We want this to change. The frustration we have felt in our clinics over a lack of time to properly address the root causes of poor health with our patients has been the main driver towards creating this guide. Since certain aspects of our modern lifestyles have caused much of the current health crisis, only addressing these factors has the potential to make a proper impact. There are of course diseases that cannot be completely cured, but even with these, addressing the same underlying factors can lessen the severity of symptoms.

The goal of this guide is to provide a starting point for lifestyle changes that will help unlock improved health and happiness. We have aimed to create a concise, practical approach with simple steps that can be implemented immediately, the positive effects of which can be felt within a matter of days. The advice we offer equally applies to healthy people who have no medical conditions, since most people want to optimise how they feel right now, and reduce the risk of developing problems in the future. We are unable to simply recommend the latest public health advice since it often fails to give enough weight to the underlying causes of the modern health crisis, and sometimes offers out of date or incorrect advice.

We will propose ten lifestyle tips that we believe will help you to achieve better health. First, a basic understanding of the theory that underpins these tips is given, covering ten key topics. The information and advice given in this guide is based on years of patient interaction and feedback, reading of up to date literature, and our family's passion for a healthy lifestyle.

Options for more in depth reading will be given at the end. Our focus will be on brevity and practical application.

Our ultimate goal is to help people feel better, both physically and mentally, and give people the knowledge and tools to empower them to improve their own health, whilst also setting healthy patterns for future generations. We want people to be less reliant on pharmaceutical companies, health care systems and doctors.

PART 1
THE THEORY

1. MODERN MEDICINE AND CHRONIC DISEASE

A lot of modern medicine involves treating the symptoms of disease, rather than addressing the root causes. Whereas this is fine for a broken arm, it is not as effective when it comes to chronic disease. Chronic disease refers to long term conditions which tend to develop as life goes on and that are rarely cured. Examples include high blood pressure, type 2 diabetes, cardiovascular disease, gastrointestinal disorders, depression and anxiety, osteoarthritis, osteoporosis, autoimmune conditions, many cancers, and dementia. The mainstay of treatment for these conditions is prescription drugs. But drugs often do a fairly poor job at managing chronic disease, and rarely provide a cure. Rather, they simply mask symptoms or mitigate some of the disease effects. These drugs, often designed to be taken for years or lifelong, are usually not solutions because they are not targeting the root causes of the diseases they aim to treat. The root causes are often to be found within common patterns of our modern lifestyles. Prevention or a cure by way of a lifestyle change makes a pharmaceutical company no money, whereas medications taken lifelong to treat ongoing disease produce big profits.

The rise of modern science and medicine has at times contributed to an arrogance that disregards the complexity of the natural world. It was thought that nature could be understood, and then controlled, without consequence. There has been a widespread failure to appreciate just how complicated and interconnected the human body and nature are, and how our best intentions to interfere often create unforeseen downstream problems including obesity, chronic disease and environmental degradation.

Modern medicine also tends to overlook the interconnectedness of the whole body. Drugs that improve symptoms in one area commonly cause problems in another, many of which are unknown to the doctor prescribing them. A reductionist mindset is often employed by the modern medical drugs based approach, with the body broken down into overly simplistic parts, and then drug therapy targeted at one of these parts. Little consideration is given to how drugs may affect other areas of the body when taken long term. Although it is useful to employ terms such as 'cardiovascular disease' and 'mental health conditions', they should not be used at the expense of realising that all parts of the body are interdependent. Stress, for example, is a direct cause of raised blood pressure and therefore cardiovascular disease. Physical health and mental health are closely related. A good example of the complexity and interconnectedness of the body is illustrated by the idea that the type of bugs living in our gut can affect our mood and mental health.

Drug therapy is unable to address this level of complexity. As a consequence, both science and modern health care often fail to provide the solutions people need to improve their overall health. But lifestyle changes can, as they enable our bodies to restore order and balance for proper functioning. Science can play a role in exploring how the body works, and so help provide an understanding of the importance of lifestyle choices, though this is often knowledge that previous generations knew instinctively. Ultimately, the way to a happy, healthy life is not, for the most part, through medicine and technology.

Whilst we cannot control all the factors in our modern lifestyles that contribute to poor health, four of the most important root causes that we have the ability to address ourselves are:

1. Poor nutrition
2. Disruption of body clocks
3. Imbalance of the autonomic nervous system
4. Poor movement patterns

These four factors drive obesity and poor health, in part by disrupting the balance of many key hormones involved in the proper functioning of the body.

2. WEIGHT REGULATION AND THE WEIGHT SET POINT

The common reason given as to why people gain weight relates to the idea of calories-in vs calories-out. According to this idea, if you take in more energy than you use up, you gain weight; if you use up more energy than you take in, you lose weight. So take in less energy by eating fewer calories, and use up more energy by exercising more, and weight loss will occur. Many people who have tried this approach have been unable to achieve lasting change to their weight.

The reason that this approach often fails is because we overestimate our ability to control the number of calories we eat and the amount of energy we expend, both of which we often believe we can manage using self control and conscious effort. Although we do have some conscious control over this calories-in vs calories-out balance, our subconscious brain has much more of an influence, and has much more powerful tools than self control at its disposal. Our brain regulates our weight using hormones, as well as by adjusting metabolic rate.

Since having either too much or too little fat causes problems with survival in the natural world, our brain aims to keep our body fat, and therefore our weight, at a constant ideal level. This is called the weight set point. To do this, the brain first needs to know how much fat we have stored. This is done using the hormone leptin, which is released by fat cells throughout the body, and sensed by the brain. The more fat we have, the more leptin we release, and so the brain can monitor if we rise above or fall below our weight set point.

If our weight falls below the weight set point during a calorie restricting diet, leptin levels decrease. The brain senses this and may perceive a threat from starvation, thinking that we have entered a famine. Hunger hormones such as ghrelin, that encourage us to seek out food, are increased, whilst fullness hormones, that help us feel full after eating, are decreased. Our metabolic rate is slowed, meaning the body uses up less energy at rest. Calorie intake therefore increases whilst energy output decreases. In this way our brain tries to push our weight back up to the weight set point.

When people who have tried a calorie restricting diet hear this, it often resonates with them. In the first week of the diet, all was going well and some weight loss occurred. But then cravings increased and they felt constantly hungry (because hunger hormones increased and fullness hormones decreased), and they felt generally fatigued and miserable (because metabolic rate slowed). They regained any lost weight and felt demoralised. In reality, no degree of self discipline could have allowed them to overcome these powerful hormonal and metabolic effects.

To add insult to injury, after a diet has ended, some people may end up heavier than when they started. This is because the lower metabolic rate and increased hunger hormones are known to persist even after a calorie restricting diet has ended. The brain doesn't want to take any chances and so is happy to increase the weight set point and store extra fat in order to be more prepared for the next famine. Repeated cycles of this, so called yo-yo dieting, compound the problem, and can drive the weight set point up. All this makes diets that focus on continuous calorie restriction counter productive.

Whilst this often makes sense to people, the opposing scenario tends not to. When the weight set point mechanisms are working properly, our brain does not just act to stop us losing fat, but also to stop us gaining excess fat. If we overeat, gaining some fat, leptin levels increase and the brain senses this. Hunger hormones are decreased, fullness hormones are increased and metabolic rate is sped up. Calorie intake therefore decreases whilst energy output increases, and the unnecessary extra fat is lost effortlessly, resulting in a return to the weight set point.

This should be the experience of people eating a healthy diet. Effortless weight control, subconsciously regulated, without the need to count calories or exercise excessively. Why then is the experience of many completely contrary to this? Why do people continue to gain weight despite their best efforts?

There are two main reasons why this may occur. The first is due to a diet composed of overly processed foods, rather than whole natural foods. Overly processed foods lack the right amount of micronutrients (vitamins, minerals and polyphenols) that the body needs. The brain therefore drives the weight set point up, not because it needs more fat reserves, but because it needs more micronutrients. Eating a higher quantity of food may be the only way to obtain a sufficient quantity of micronutrients. However, if overly processed foods continue to be consumed, micronutrient amounts are never enough, and the weight set point is driven ever upwards, causing the eater to continue gaining weight. This state is described by the phrase 'overfed but undernourished'.

The second reason that people may continue to gain weight is because their brain is no longer sensing leptin levels correctly. This means that if extra fat is gained and leptin levels rise, the brain is unaware of it, and so does not attempt to reverse the weight gain. This is called leptin resistance. Even if fat reserves and leptin levels are both increasing, leptin resistance may cause the brain to think leptin levels are low and so perceive starvation and drive the weight set point up. Two important factors that contribute to leptin resistance are excess insulin and generalised inflammation throughout the body.

To maintain a healthy weight, It is therefore crucial to eat micronutrient dense foods rather than overly processed foods, avoid excess insulin and avoid being in an inflammatory state. This will allow the brain to sense leptin properly and the body to obtain enough micronutrients, keeping the weight regulation system correctly calibrated. Our subconscious brain can then take care of the calories-in vs calories-out balance, tipping the equation when needed by adjusting our hunger and metabolism in order to keep us at, or return us to, a healthy weight.

3. INSULIN

Insulin is the body's main storage hormone. In response to raised blood glucose (blood sugar) levels after eating, insulin rises in order to remove excess glucose from the bloodstream. This acts to keep blood glucose concentration at a safe level and store away the energy from glucose for later use. Glucose is first stored as glycogen in the liver and muscle, and once glycogen stores are full, glucose is taken up by cells that convert it and store the energy as fat. Elevated insulin puts the body into storage mode. Low insulin levels that occur when we are not eating allow the body to bring energy out of storage to use for fuel between meals.

Consistently high insulin levels keep the body in storage mode and can contribute to leptin resistance because the high insulin level can block the brain's ability to sense leptin properly. Consistently high insulin is the most significant driver of obesity. How high insulin levels go after eating is determined by the type of food eaten. How often this happens is determined by how often food is eaten throughout each 24 hour day.

Consistently high levels of insulin also cause another major problem: insulin resistance. Just like some people experience caffeine tolerance, with high exposure to caffeine leading to higher doses being needed to get the same effect, consistently high levels of insulin lead to insulin resistance, with the body needing higher levels of insulin than before to get the same effect in regulating blood glucose levels. A vicious cycle is easily entered. Excessive insulin levels drive both weight gain and insulin resistance, which in turn leads to even higher insulin levels.

Insulin resistance is implicated as a main cause of chronic disease. This spans problems from cardiovascular disease and fatty liver disease, to dementia and migraines, to reproductive health problems such as polycystic ovarian syndrome (PCOS) in women and low testosterone in men, as well as cancers including breast and prostate, skin conditions including acne and psoriasis, and many more. Insulin resistance drives both obesity and chronic disease.

Type 2 diabetes occurs when the degree of insulin resistance is so high that despite high insulin levels, there is inadequate control of blood glucose levels. However, a lower but very significant degree of insulin resistance is prevalent in many people with completely normal blood glucose levels, well before even prediabetes (the precursor to type 2 diabetes) kicks in. High insulin levels, even in those with normal blood glucose readings, are a major driver of chronic disease. But doctors don't generally measure blood insulin, only blood glucose, and may give out false reassurance based on normal blood glucose results.

It is in everyone's best interest to avoid excess insulin levels and subsequent insulin resistance, and instead remain in a healthy insulin sensitive state. The good news is that insulin is a hormone that we can influence with conscious effort, by altering the type of food we consume and the pattern of how we consume it, alongside other lifestyle interventions. Insulin resistance can be reversed. Our ability to influence insulin, combined with its central role in chronic disease, makes reducing insulin levels and avoiding insulin resistance a good place to start when it comes to improving health.

4. CARBOHYDRATES

The main macronutrient food groups are fat, protein, and carbohydrate. Carbohydrates (starch and sugar) are a significant energy source, and the most important macronutrient to consider when it comes to insulin. Starches are long chains of glucose units joined together. Table sugar (sucrose) is one glucose unit and one fructose unit joined together. After we eat, the absorption of glucose from carbohydrates in food is the main driver of insulin secretion.

When eaten in isolation, both starch and sugar are rapidly digested in the gut producing individual glucose units that are then absorbed into the bloodstream. This causes a rapid spike in blood glucose levels. In response, a high level of insulin is secreted into the bloodstream. This high insulin response causes a sudden reduction in blood glucose levels, quickly reversing the initial blood glucose spike. This rapid change in blood glucose levels can sap people of energy and stimulate hunger again quickly, particularly driving a craving for more glucose-containing carbohydrates. The higher the glucose spike after food, the quicker hunger returns. This can lead to a cycle of regular snacking on starchy or sugary products, resulting in consistently high levels of insulin. Snacking culture has become normalised in society today, but in time it often leads to insulin resistance.

There is an additional problem with sugar when compared with starch. Since sugar also contains fructose, when sugar is consumed in isolation there is a corresponding fructose spike along with the glucose spike. Whereas glucose provides immediate energy, fructose does not. The liver has to deal with fructose in a similar way to alcohol. Although a fructose spike does not induce an insulin response, if the liver is overwhelmed by an excess amount of fructose, liver fat accumulation and liver inflammation can occur, just as happens with excess alcohol intake. Non-alcoholic fatty liver disease (NAFLD) can occur, an increasingly common finding in adults, and now even children. Fatty liver disease drives further insulin resistance, and is itself strongly associated with the development of many chronic health conditions. Excess fructose also has negative effects elsewhere including the brain, likely contributing to behavioural issues in children and cognitive impairment in the elderly. This all makes excess sugar consumption a bigger problem than excess starch consumption.

Following the increased recognition of the health implications of regular spikes in blood glucose, fructose and insulin, a lot of blame has been attributed to carbohydrates. Low carbohydrate diets have gained popularity. These diets aid weight loss by reducing insulin levels. Reducing levels of the storage hormone allows weight loss, and insulin sensitivity can be regained. These low carbohydrate diets are useful in some circumstances and as treatment for certain conditions. They can be used as a healthy lifestyle choice for those who find they do well on them. For many people however, low carbohydrate diets can be hard to persevere with. Also, population centres around the world that have been identified as having above average lifespans and low rates of chronic disease, the so-called blue zones (which include areas in the Mediterranean), often have moderate to high levels of carbohydrate in their diets. One common feature shared by residents inhabiting blue zones is an unprocessed diet, and it is nature that provides the antidote for any problems posed by carbohydrates.

In whole unprocessed foods, carbohydrates (both sugar and starch), do not occur in isolation, but come with other components, such as fibre, that slow the digestion and the absorption of starch and sugar, reducing the problem of sudden spikes in blood glucose, fructose and insulin. Like starch, fibre is also simply long chains of glucose units joined together. However, unlike starch, our digestive enzymes cannot break down the type of chain links in fibre, and so the glucose is not made available for absorption. Fibre, fat and protein all slow down, to varying degrees, the digestion of starch and sugar and their absorption into the bloodstream. Fibre in particular seems to be nature's antidote to any problematic spikes, with its ability to physically block and slow down both digestion and absorption of carbohydrates.

Overly processed foods have often had fibre and micronutrients stripped from them during processing. This is one of the key differences between unprocessed whole foods, such as nuts and fruit, and overly processed foods, such as table sugar and white flour. It is the processing that results in naturally occurring components of healthy whole foods, such as glucose and fructose, suddenly becoming major health concerns when consumed excessively in relative isolation, without sufficient protective factors such as fibre. The lack of micronutrients in overly processed foods also contributes to excess intake. This is in addition to the fact that they are less effective at stimulating fullness hormones, a further factor in overconsumption. Carbohydrates as a whole are not the problem. It is overly processed carbohydrates, especially table sugar (due to its fructose content), that drive poor health. Low fibre, low micronutrient carbohydrates are a major health concern.

The glycaemic index (GI) diet attempts to limit foods that cause big glucose spikes, but classifying foods based solely on their effect on blood glucose has a number of flaws. It does not take into account fructose, and gives no information about the overall nutritional quality of the food, as it does not consider micronutrient content or whether a food may cause negative health impacts elsewhere, as is the case with artificial sweeteners. Some artificial sweeteners even cause an insulin response, with the body acting to preempt the expected glucose arrival after the tongue detects a sweet taste, even if no glucose arrives.

Another approach to carbohydrates is to check the nutritional information label in order to compare the amount of carbohydrate per 100g to the amount of fibre per 100g, and so avoid foods that have a high carbohydrate:fibre ratio (these foods are often referred to as 'starchy'). This might drive a preference for legumes such as black beans or lentils (starch and fibre content roughly equal) over potatoes (ten times as much starch than fibre). Comparing like with like, for example two loaves of bread, may be a more useful exercise. However, in a balanced food plate with plenty of other fibre rich vegetables, the carbohydrate:fibre ratio of any one food should become a relatively minor issue. Maximising the variety of whole foods, rather than adding restrictions, is usually the best approach for good health.

We want to avoid falling into the trap of nutritional reductionism, where we judge a food in an overly simplistic manner, based solely on one characteristic. Whereas this does work for overly processed foods which have often been stripped down to basic components, whole minimally processed foods are complex and contain many other components, such as micronutrients, which contribute to the overall picture of how healthy they are. It is best to avoid restricting unprocessed whole foods and instead focus on eliminating overly processed ones. Stick to food that resembles how it appears in nature, in the context of a balanced plate and good eating patterns, and the problems associated with overly processed carbohydrates can be eliminated.

5. INFLAMMATION

There is now increasing recognition that many disease processes involve chronic inflammation. This is well known for certain diseases traditionally understood as being inflammatory, such as inflammatory bowel disease or rheumatoid arthritis. But now other conditions, such as cardiovascular disease and cancers, are recognised as being driven in part by chronic inflammation. Short lived inflammation in a localised area of the body, as happens with an injury or during an infection, is a helpful response. The problem lies in long standing levels of widespread generalised inflammation throughout the body. High blood levels of glucose and fructose cause inflammation. Fasting is an important tool in reducing chronic inflammation. Polyphenols are beneficial plant compounds often found in colourful plants. Polyphenol rich foods such as cacao, berries, red wine, nuts, seeds, herbs, spices, olives and coffee, are thought to reduce inflammation.

Dietary fat, whilst having minimal effect on stimulating insulin secretion, is also important to consider when it comes to inflammation. Omega-3 polyunsaturated fats are important dietary fats that have anti-inflammatory effects. The especially healthy long chain omega-3s are found in fish, wild or grass fed meats, and eggs. Long chain omega-3s are important for brain health, and are thought to help conditions including cardiovascular disease, eye disease and depression. Medium chain omega-3s are found in high amounts in certain plant foods such as flax and chia seed, however the body is not always efficient at converting them to long chain omega-3s.

A modern overly processed diet tends to have a low intake of omega-3s, but a high intake of omega-6 polyunsaturated fats. Excess consumption of omega-6s may have pro-inflammatory effects, and there is increasing interest in the omega 3 to omega 6 ratio in the modern western diet. In an unprocessed diet, the consumption ratio of omega 3 to omega 6 may approach 1:1. These omega fats are incorporated into the cells throughout our body in the same ratio as they are consumed in, and influence cell function. Roughly equal proportions of pro-inflammatory elements and anti-inflammatory elements create a healthy balance. However, the omega 3:6 ratio in a modern diet may be more like 1:20, due to an under consumption of omega-3s and a high consumption of omega-6s. This may contribute to pro-inflammatory conditions throughout the body. Generalised inflammation can affect the brain's ability to sense leptin, contributing to leptin resistance and obesity. Excess body fat itself causes further generalised inflammation creating a vicious cycle.

Omega-6s are found in nuts and seeds in high quantities. But whole nuts and seeds are healthy micronutrient dense foods, associated with reduced cardiovascular disease risk and healthy weight regulation, and they come packaged with micronutrients that protect against inflammation. Whole nuts and seeds are clearly not the problem: in fact unprocessed whole foods are never the problem.

Instead, highly processed oils derived from seeds such as sunflower oil, rapeseed oil (canola oil) and vegetable oil are likely to be problematic. These seed oils only became a major player in human diets in the 20th century, since they require significant industrial and chemical processing to produce, during which the health giving properties and micronutrients of the seeds are mostly lost. Seed oils are found everywhere in supermarkets, restaurants and fast food, facilitating a high intake of overly processed omega-6s, and a significant change in the omega 3:6 ratio in a typical modern western diet.

Additionally, polyunsaturated fats, including omega-6s, are the most unstable type of fat (saturated fat being the most stable, monounsaturated fats such as in extra virgin olive oil being the next most stable). Stability in this case refers to how well they fare at resisting degradation and oxidation once outside their natural housing. In the case of polyunsaturated fats, including omega-6s, it turns out they fare badly once removed from the nut or seed that they come from, especially after industrial processing, which further increases their potential to contribute to a pro-inflammatory state once consumed.

Incredibly, overly processed polyunsaturated fats in seed oils continue to be promoted as heart healthy foods in public health messaging. Cheap highly processed oils that permeate junk food, and that only entered our diet in the 20th century, seem an unlikely candidate for a healthy food.

In a classic case of nutritional reductionism, public health messaging during the later half of the 20th century instead chose saturated fat as the scapegoat for the emerging health crisis. This was regardless of the quality of food it was contained in or the level of processing it had been through. The decision to blame saturated fat was in part based on dubious conclusions drawn from notoriously unreliable correlation studies, often funded by the sugar industry. As a result, public health messaging drove people towards consuming more overly processed grain and sugar, the very foods fueling the health crisis.

For the first time in human history low fat diets were perceived as desirable. Saturated fat has always been a staple of human nutrition, including in food such as liver that has been recognised as one of the most nutrient dense foods available throughout human history. The Hadza, a modern day hunter-gatherer people in Tanzania, prize organ meat. Unsurprisingly, they are not affected by the chronic diseases that modern nutrition and lifestyle inflict. There is no one type of fat that is inherently bad for humans. Rather it is the overly processed ones, of which seed oils are a prime example, that contribute to chronic disease and obesity. It has also become increasingly clear that it is insulin resistance, rather than saturated fat or dietary cholesterol intake, that leads to unhealthy blood cholesterol profiles.

In the case of animal fats and animal products more generally, the quality of life experienced by the animal impacts the nutritional benefits of the food. Intensively farmed animals, including farmed fish, have a miserable lifestyle and poor nutrition. The feeds they are given commonly contain overly processed grains and seed oils, and they often end up consuming large quantities of antibiotics, and in some countries synthetic hormones. This results in poor quality food. Wild fish, wild meats and well looked after farm animals, all of which are allowed to consume their natural diet and live a more healthy active lifestyle, produce better quality food. As a result, they possess higher levels of omega-3s and micronutrients. The problem with poor quality animal products is often compounded by a higher level of processing. In this way, the nutritional profile of animal products is directly related to the nutrition and lifestyle of the animals they come from.

It should also be stressed that eating a higher proportion of fat, which is more calorie dense, does not cause people to put on weight. The calorie density of foods does not confuse the body's weight regulation system. Many calorie dense foods, such as whole nuts and full fat dairy products, are associated with good weight control and good health. The increased fat content of unprocessed fatty foods tend to contribute to a feeling of fullness, and many unprocessed fatty foods are some of the most micronutrient dense foods available. Since many vitamins are fat soluble, there is better absorption of the vitamins in foods such as vegetables when they are consumed with fat.

As in the case of carbohydrates, it seems unlikely that there is any whole unprocessed food that is inherently bad for us, and this applies to all types of fat. Rather, it is the quality and level of processing that determines whether a fat is good or bad for our health. Whole nuts and seeds are good for health; highly processed seed oils are not. High quality extra virgin olive oil, which is known for its anti-inflammatory properties, is a healthy food; overly processed and deodorised olive oil is best avoided. Raw cacao nibs, high in saturated fat and micronutrient dense, are healthy; overly processed milk chocolate, high in sugar, is not. Liver from a wild animal is good; liver from a battery animal is not. It is overly processed foods, and consuming products from animals fed them, that cause the problem.

6. THE GUT MICROBIOME

The gut microbiome is the community of bugs, mostly bacteria, that live in our gut. We are all covered head to toe in bacteria, with bugs living on our skin, in our gut and at other sites, such as the eyes, ears, mouth, nose, lungs, and vagina. Although bacteria are often associated with infectious diseases and being unwell, the vast majority of those living on and in us are important in maintaining good health. In recent years, it has become increasingly understood that a healthy gut microbiome is a major contributor to good health, both locally in the gut, and throughout the rest of the body. When considering nutrition, it is good to be aware that we are not just feeding ourselves, but also our resident gut bugs.

A healthy gut microbiome refers to a gut colonised by a wide range of beneficial, health promoting bugs. These bugs feed on the food that we eat, and support the health of our gut and many other systems in the body. A large proportion of the immune system is found at the gut, and a healthy gut microbiome is essential for a correctly working immune system. The gut microbiome also directly impacts mental health and brain function via the gut-brain axis, a two way link between the gut and the brain.

An unhealthy gut microbiome consists of an imbalanced bug population, with less beneficial bugs and more harmful bugs. This can increase the risk of developing gut problems such as IBS (irritable bowel syndrome), bowel cancer, and inflammation of the gut wall. Inflammation of the gut wall can cause increased intestinal permeability (sometimes referred to as leaky gut) which is thought to increase the risk of developing autoimmune diseases and allergies. Throughout the rest of the body, an unhealthy gut microbiome can increase insulin resistance, increase inflammation, increase susceptibility to infections, and contribute to mental health problems and behavioural issues.

The relationship between humans and their gut microbiomes is symbiotic, meaning that both parties benefit. What is good for our gut microbiome is also good for our health, and vice versa. Whilst we have enjoyed some of the changes that advancements in technology and science have brought us, our gut microbiomes have not.

The foundation for the gut microbiome is set during pregnancy. The mother's vaginal microbiome changes towards the later stages of pregnancy in order to get ready to deliver beneficial bugs to the baby. As the baby comes down the birth canal, it is coated in these bugs, which then travel to the gut and establish the newborn's gut microbiome. Babies born via C-section may instead be colonised by bacteria found in hospitals or on the skin of hospital staff. Breast milk continues to provide important support for the development of a healthy gut microbiome. Benefits of breastfeeding for the mother include improved insulin sensitivity and a reduced risk of breast cancer. In addition, sucking milk from the breast, rather than a bottle, works the baby's facial muscles, contributing to proper oral and nasal cavity development and subsequent dental alignment. At weaning, proper nutrition continues to support a child's gut microbiome (and foods that require chewing, in contrast to pureed foods, keep the facial muscles working for proper development).

Growing up in ever cleaner environments is detrimental to our resident bacteria, which are damaged by antibacterial cleaning products and household chemical cleaning sprays. The problem with overly clean environments is also linked to the hygiene hypothesis, the idea that the developing immune system requires plenty of exposure to certain bugs, and that children that lack this exposure risk getting immune system dysfunction. Ingesting chemicals, as occurs when eating food sprayed with pesticides such as glyphosate, causes harm to the gut microbiome, as do plastics and pollutants. Many pesticides, plastics and pollutants are known to be endocrine disruptors, meaning they have a direct impact on hormone systems, especially the sex hormones oestrogen and testosterone. Eating artificial ingredients such as sweeteners, flavourings, preservatives and emulsifiers all negatively impact the gut microbiome. Artificial sweeteners can even alter the microbiome in a way that goes on to contribute to insulin resistance. Medications used to treat chronic diseases often negatively impact the gut microbiome, as can contraceptive pills. To our resident bacteria, the use of antibiotics represents an indiscriminate bombing raid. Because of the effect on the gut microbiome, and subsequently the gut brain-axis, taking antibiotics can increase the risk of developing depression and anxiety.

Considering all this, we can see why many factors in modern lifestyles are associated with a less healthy gut microbiome and subsequent immune dysregulation, giving an increased risk of developing allergies, autoimmune disease, and atopic conditions such as asthma and eczema. Later in life, a less healthy gut microbiome is associated with an increased risk of developing obesity and type 2 diabetes.

No matter what our start in life, we all have considerable influence over the health of the gut microbiome in our day to day decisions. Factors thought to be associated with a healthy gut microbiome include: maximising the variety of whole nutritious foods consumed; avoiding overly processed foods, artificial sweeteners and additives; a sufficient overnight fast each day; good exercise levels; low stress levels; good sleep quality; time interacting outdoors with nature including with animals, plants and soil; and minimising exposure to antibiotics, cleaning products, pesticides, plastics, man made chemicals and pollutants. In short, sticking as close to the way nature intended us to live as possible.

With the increased awareness of the gut microbiome has come increased interest in prebiotics and probiotics. Prebiotics are foods that provide beneficial fuel for supporting a healthy gut microbiome. Fibre, which we cannot digest and instead travels intact to our gut bugs, is thought to be a good prebiotic.

Beneficial bacteria ferment fibre, producing compounds that contribute to gut health and metabolic health.

Probiotics are foods that contain live bugs thought to be beneficial for our gut microbiome, either by direct interaction between the bugs in the food and the gut microbiome, or by the beneficial changes these bugs make to the food that contains them, or both. Examples of probiotics include live yoghurt, certain cheeses and sauerkraut. The live lactic acid bacteria in these foods use lactic acid fermentation to produce energy from the sugars in the food. This lacto-fermentation creates healthy byproducts and increases the availability of micronutrients. Unlike modern bread production involving packaged yeast, sourdough bread undergoes lacto-fermentation by bacteria, providing health benefits even after the bacteria are killed off during baking. Cheese production has long been used to circumvent the problem of lactose intolerance, with the long fermentation period involved in producing mature cheese causing the bacteria to use up all the available lactose, rendering the product virtually lactose free. Other common food fermentation processes include yeasts fermenting sugars to produce alcohol, and acetic acid bacteria fermenting alcohol to produce vinegar.

A healthy gut microbiome is best supported by a wide range of different whole foods, and both prebiotics and probiotics can contribute to this. However, the beneficial impacts we can impart to our resident gut bugs go well beyond just nutritional choices.

7. BODY CLOCKS

Many of our organs are now known to have an innate ability to keep time. The mechanisms by which cells and organs keep time are referred to as body clocks. Organs need clocks for much the same reason we do, in order to structure the day and make sure enough time is allocated to each necessary task. For example, the gut has a clock so that it can schedule time for digestion and moving food through the gut efficiently, as well as time for rest and repair. The clocks in each organ naturally keep time to a daily cycle of close to 24 hours. Biological rhythms that follow 24 hour cycles are called circadian rhythms.

There is a master clock in the brain which helps to coordinate all the different clocks throughout the body to run in sync. This is important because there is little point in the gut being in the rest and repair phase during the day time when we are planning to eat. The coordination of body clocks is vital for proper functioning of each organ. As well as coordinating different body clocks to one another, the master clock also syncs the clocks and biological functions throughout the body to the natural day-night cycle. The master clock receives information from the eyes about when it is light, and therefore day time, and when it is dark, and therefore night time.

In a natural environment, early morning light falling on the eye signals to the master clock that it is morning. There is a morning spike in cortisol, a hormone contributing to alertness and preparing the body for the day ahead. This wakes up other organs, such as the gut, preparing them for daytime tasks. Cortisol declines during daylight hours, reaching a low in the evening at bedtime. As the brain senses lower levels of light in the evening, the hormone melatonin increases, eventually triggering the desire to sleep. Cortisol and melatonin are examples of hormones that follow a circadian rhythm, with peaks and dips in their levels at certain times in each 24 hour cycle.

Many patterns in modern living do well at disrupting body clocks and normal circadian rhythms. A lack of time outdoors throughout the day, particularly the morning, reduces exposure to sunlight and begins the disruption of the master clock. A reduction of early bright daylight exposure means that melatonin can persist into the morning, and the early spike in cortisol may be delayed, both of which reduce morning alertness. Breakfast may be consumed before the gut has had its wake up call. A stressful sedentary day can lead to high evening cortisol levels, disrupting the relaxed state needed to generate sleep. The normal circadian rhythm of cortisol is disrupted in many mental health conditions including depression, ADHD and autism. Once one hormone in a complex system is dysregulated, others (such as dopamine and serotonin) tend to follow.

Artificial lighting after dark, as well as light from TV, computer, and phone screens, disrupts melatonin production. Along with the stimulation created by these devices, this increases evening alertness, encouraging a late bedtime. Many people who feel they naturally go to bed late and do well on this schedule have in fact artificially shifted their sleep-wake cycle by means of evening exposure to artificial lighting and screens.

Good sleep at the correct time of day sits at the centre of properly coordinated body clocks and healthy circadian rhythms. Good levels of melatonin at night contribute to a deep restorative sleep. Since sleep is the primary way the body undergoes restoration and repair, it follows that poor sleep will impact every aspect of physical and mental health and wellbeing. Even people who feel they fall asleep perfectly well after looking at screens late at night will have the amount of melatonin they produce reduced, worsening the quality of their sleep and leading to reduced energy levels the following day. As well as being involved in coordinating sleep, melatonin plays an important role in reducing inflammation and regulating the immune system, and is important for bone health and helping reduce the risk of osteoporosis. Poor sleep also directly contributes to insulin resistance and increases levels of the hunger hormone ghrelin.

The gut expects to be working to process food for approximately 10 hours during the day, and then get a significant rest overnight. The gut clock wants to be in sync with the main clock in the brain, digesting food during the light of the day and resting during the darkness of night. The body is much more efficient at metabolising the energy provided by digestion of food during the day, and melatonin reduces the efficiency of metabolism at night. Modern lifestyle patterns often involve eating throughout an extended portion of the 24 hour day, starting very soon after waking and continuing late into the evening, disrupting the gut circadian rhythm and compromising the body's ability to process food efficiently. An inadequate rest period without food overnight can contribute to many gut problems. The stomach produces more acid in response to meals consumed late in the evening compared to meals eaten earlier in the day, due to the circadian rhythm in stomach acid production. This consequence of late eating, combined with less efficient gastric emptying in the evening, as well as lying flat too soon after food when eating late, are often factors in acid reflux and indigestion.

Caffeine and alcohol intake can disrupt circadian rhythms and sleep. Although alcohol may help people fall asleep quickly, this is because it is a sedative, and rather than inducing natural sleep, this actually worsens sleep quality. Caffeine consumed in the later part of the day also impacts the quality of sleep. Some medications can also cause disruption, as is the case with beta-blockers (prescribed commonly for those with cardiovascular disease or anxiety) which can significantly reduce melatonin production. Good sleep can be gauged by feeling well rested and alert on waking, without the need to rely on stimulants such as caffeine to function optimally.

Similar to jet lag, all these disruptions create confusion for the master clock and other body clocks, with the master clock out of sync with natural daylight, and other body clocks out of sync with each other. This causes strain on many systems and contributes to inflammation throughout the body. It is therefore no surprise that the disruption of body clocks and circadian rhythms is increasingly being recognised as an important factor in chronic disease. Although sleep sits at the centre of good circadian rhythm, the measures needed to optimise our body's natural rhythms are influenced by our choices throughout the day, starting first thing in the morning.

8. THE AUTONOMIC NERVOUS SYSTEM

The autonomic nervous system regulates key processes in the body such as heart rate, breathing rate, blood pressure, and digestion. The autonomic nervous system is divided into the sympathetic nervous system and the parasympathetic nervous system. The parasympathetic nervous system is responsible for rest-and-digest mode, a relaxed state characterised by a normally low blood pressure, pulse rate and breathing rate, with a focus on normal organ activities, such as digestion, running smoothly and efficiently. If a sudden dangerous situation were to present itself, such as coming face to face with a pack of hungry wolves, the sympathetic nervous system activates the fight-or-flight response, causing the release of adrenaline and cortisol. These hormones trigger an increase in blood pressure, pulse rate, breathing rate, and blood glucose concentration. These are all useful and necessary measures needed for the sudden burst of intense activity needed to run away. Energy is diverted away from any unnecessary functions, such as digestion. Once the threat is over, the fight-or-flight response can be switched off and rest-and-digest mode restarted.

The balance between the activation of these two arms of the autonomic nervous system is important for good health.

Rest-and-digest is the mode we should live almost all of each day in. The fight-or-flight response is designed as a short lived and infrequently experienced state. Unfortunately, many people have an imbalance in the activation of these two states, and spend significant portions of the day in a low grade fight-or-flight response. This is because the psychological stresses of the modern world, be it work or school, financial concerns, relationship problems, or even factors such as running late, frustration at being stuck in traffic, concern over popularity on social media, reading the news, a cluttered house, being too busy or having a long to-do list, can all elicit a low grade but significant activation of the sympathetic nervous system.

Apart from a general feeling of anxiety, excessive time spent in a fight-or-flight response contributes to high blood pressure and cardiovascular disease, raised blood glucose and subsequent insulin resistance, and a host of digestive problems including IBS. For many people, prolonged elevation of cortisol increases hunger and the weight set point, leading to weight gain. Prolonged elevation of cortisol can cause disruption of other hormones, with a reduction in oestrogen levels in women and testosterone levels in men. Prolonged activation of the fight-or-flight response increases susceptibility to infection, and is associated with generalised chronic inflammation. The normal circadian rhythm of cortisol is also disrupted, with elevated evening cortisol levels disrupting sleep, which in turn causes further cortisol elevation. This exhausts the body and depletes the individual of energy. Attempting to subdue stress through excess alcohol intake also increases cortisol levels.

Excessive time spent in a fight-or-flight response can also reduce the speed and ease at which the body can switch back into rest-and-digest mode. Tools are therefore often needed to release people from a fight-or-flight state. Passive measures that people tend to think will help, such as slumping in front of the TV with a beer after a stressful day, often turn out to be a pretty ineffective solution. Moving out of a fight-or-flight state, which in effect means stress relief, is an active process.

For quick short term stress relief, exercise is an effective tool. In a fight-or-flight response, the body is anticipating a burst of physical activity. Exercise gives it this, helping to burn off some of the nervous energy associated with this state, and so aiding an efficient return to rest-and-digest mode. This can be done quickly, with just a 60 second burst of intense physical activity being effective in some cases. Less intensive activity such as going for a walk can also be effective.

Exercise is an example of hormetic stress. Hormetic stress refers to a short burst of beneficial stress that encourages the body to adapt in order to become more resilient. These self induced stressful activities often cause a temporary activation of the flight-or-fight response, but once stopped they efficiently transition the user into rest-and-digest mode. Hormetic stress is very different from psychological stress when it comes to the effects on the body and mind, promoting beneficial responses and usually resulting in a sense of satisfaction and achievement due to the release of endorphins. Other forms of hormetic stress include cold exposure (such as cold water swimming), heat exposure (such as a sauna) and fasting. Regular exposure to hormetic stress improves both physical and mental resilience, and trains the body to be more efficient at transitioning back into rest-and-digest mode after psychological stress. In this way, a burst of exercise provides a quick aid to a stressful day whilst regular exercise allows people to become more stress resilient.

Breathing exercises are another tool for stress relief which work by helping to activate rest-and-digest mode. Unlike blood pressure, pulse rate or cortisol secretion, which are out of our control, breathing patterns are something regulated by the autonomic nervous system that we can consciously alter immediately. Conscious alteration of breathing patterns away from those characteristic of a fight-or-flight response, and towards those characteristic of rest-and-digest mode, can effectively cause the transition to take place. In a fight-or-flight response, breathing is typically fast and shallow, using expansion of the upper chest to draw breath into the lungs through the mouth. In rest-and-digest mode, breathing is slower and done through the nose, expanding the belly to draw the breath in, which means engaging the diaphragm at the base of the lungs, rather than chest muscles. Knowing these patterns can make us aware of how to breathe in order to help reduce fight-or-flight activation, by consciously slowing our breathing rate, and engaging the belly to breathe in and out through the nose. An awareness of breathing patterns sits at the core of many stress-targeting activities such as yoga and meditation.

Belly and nasal breathing come with other notable health advantages. Diaphragm movement creates pressure changes in the abdomen, contributing to blood circulation and taking some of the workload off the heart. Because of this, the diaphragm is sometimes referred to as the second heart. As opposed to mouth breathing, nasal breathing filters some pollutants and harmful bugs, as well as humidifying and warming air before it enters the lungs. Nasal breathing also causes the release of nitric oxide which acts to dilate blood vessels and aid blood circulation throughout the body. Mouth breathing can negatively impact the balance of bacteria in the mouth, whereas nasal breathing helps support a healthy oral microbiome, improving dental hygiene. In children, mouth breathing negatively impacts the proper development of the jaw and facial bones, leading to dental alignment problems.

Given that excessive time in a fight-or-flight state and consistently high levels of cortisol are key drivers in chronic health problems and obesity, it is important to address stress. Methods to help turn off the fight-or-flight response are useful, but ultimately the root causes triggering stress in the first place require careful consideration. Many life stresses may feel as though they are somewhat inevitable, such as the pressure of work required to earn enough money to pay the bills. Whilst true, there also seem to be significant stresses associated with modern lifestyles that can be mitigated.

Often, much money is spent on non-essential items pushed as necessary by social trends and advertising. These could include a TV, a TV licence, a subscription to a movie streaming service, the latest smartphone or computer, a more expensive car, new kitchen gadgets, the current fashion trends, an excess of childrens toys, expensive days out, and eating and drinking out. Money spent on many other non-essential material goods, and the subsequent clutter they usually create, can all contribute to stress, and many of them contribute in other ways to worsening physical and mental health. Being content to live with less can bring more freedom.

Social media, and much of the content promoted on it, is clearly having quite a detrimental effect on many people, especially children in whom it can fuel mental health problems. The increased importance placed on the superficial has led people away from discovering deeper purpose in life. The high prevalence of mental health conditions gives testimony to the idea that modern values and lifestyles often fail to deliver fulfilling lives. Being constantly busy is often used to distract our attention away from this problem, and it also prevents us from addressing these issues.

Consumerism and materialism appear to worsen health and mood. Screens and social media also appear to make people more unhealthy and more unhappy, as does having the pursuit of comfort and money as the main purpose of life. When society as a whole is unhealthy, both mentally and physically, it becomes necessary to break with societal norms in order to obtain good health. Feeling the need to fit into societal norms, even when they cause more harm than good, tends to come from a position of insecurity. This insecurity often stems from a lack of support that only deep family or community relationships can provide, both of which modern society has eroded. Time diverted away from superficial relationships that social media encourages and towards deep and meaningful family and community relationships is therefore an important foundation from which to combat stress.

A life full of deep purpose is able to inspire choosing a different path to that promoted by modern society. A life without deep meaning promotes superficial concerns that add to stress. Population centres with low rates of chronic disease (the blue zones) tend to have close knit supportive communities and a shared sense of purpose, which both contribute to longevity. It is important to think about purpose in life, along with considering which factors are helping to achieve that purpose, and which factors are getting in the way. This is no small task, and requires time away from the busyness of life and the distraction of screens in order to allow a careful assessment.

9. MOVEMENT

Exercise is a hormetic stress used to strengthen the body. Most people are familiar with the many benefits that it brings including improvements in cardiovascular fitness, muscle strength, joint health, sleep, and mental health. Exercise plays an important role in improving insulin sensitivity and normalising cortisol levels.

At the actual time of exercise, the hormetic stress occurring means cortisol levels can rise. However the net effect following exercise is a reduction in cortisol levels and the normalisation of the circadian rhythm of cortisol. To avoid a spike in cortisol too close to bedtime, it is advisable not to do strenuous exercise late in the evening as this could disturb sleep.

Whilst both endurance and strength training are important for good health, these activities account for a relatively brief period of time. At least as much attention, if not more, should be given to movement patterns during the rest of the day. These movement patterns are referred to as non-exercise activity, and include any activity that requires physical effort but is not intense enough to induce a hormetic stress. This could include walking, housework or a leisurely bike ride. Patterns of non-exercise activity have changed significantly over recent decades, with less time throughout the day spent walking and moving, and more time spent sitting in chairs.

Being sedentary reduces insulin sensitivity and increases the risk for almost every physical and mental health problem, including obesity, type 2 diabetes, cancer, cardiovascular disease and depression. Another casualty in a sedentary life are our backs, which suffer from the muscle imbalances that occur from prolonged chair sitting and lack of movement. Chairs tend to inactivate and weaken the glutes (buttock muscles), a key core muscle group, the neglect of which impacts many back and knee complaints. Incorporating glute specific exercises into a weekly exercise routine is often needed in order to switch on and strengthen this important but often neglected muscle group. Prolonged sitting also worsens posture and can cause neck and shoulder pain.

Another group of muscles that has been impacted by modern trends are the muscles in our feet. Modern shoes that provide excessive cushioning and support have inactivated and weakened foot muscles, causing muscle weakness issues such as collapsed arches, and predisposing us to a range of foot conditions including plantar fasciitis. The way people walk and run has been completely changed, with cushioning allowing high impact movement that transmits excessive force to knees, hips and back. The alignment of all these joints has been affected by the almost universal heel elevation in modern footwear which sets an unnatural structural foundation for the body. Many joint issues are caused by or worsened because of what we are doing at ground level. Unnaturally shaped modern footwear which crushes the toes together has led to deformities such as bunions becoming widespread. Fortunately, minimalist footwear is becoming more available as people recognise the problems we have been causing ourselves.

Regular movement throughout the day helps avoid the problems associated with a sedentary lifestyle, as well as helping manage stress, increase energy, improve focus, improve sleep, and increase insulin sensitivity. Non-exercise activity after a meal, such as going for a walk, has a dramatic effect on the insulin response needed to deal with the incoming glucose that occurs after eating. Moving muscles start to use up glucose from the meal as it appears in the bloodstream, without the need for insulin. This leaves less available glucose from the meal and so less insulin is required to deal with the remainder. Going for a walk after eating is therefore an effective step in improving insulin sensitivity, and a pleasant way to finish a meal.

Without regular movement throughout the day, both mental and physical health will inevitably suffer. In children, insufficient daily movement and exercise can cause or worsen behavioural issues. Getting outside into nature is a great place for movement to take place, giving the additional benefits of fresh air, improvements in the gut microbiome, vitamin D production, and the positive mental health aspects that immersion in nature brings. It is important to aim to move as much as possible throughout the entire day and avoid prolonged time in chairs and sofas.

10. PROCESSED LIVING

Now that we have considered several important factors impacting health, we can start to understand what has been going wrong in the modern world. Food became increasingly processed in the 20th century, and poor dietary advice led to a shift away from micronutrient dense whole foods, and towards the consumption of overly processed grains, seed oils and sugar. Whilst fibre and micronutrients were being stripped from food during processing, a multitude of artificial non-food ingredients were being added. Crops were selectively bred, becoming increasingly reliant on high levels of pesticides and chemical fertilisers, damaging ecosystems and causing soil degradation. Intensive farming practices increased. Microplastics appeared in food. Many contaminants entered the drinking water supply, including synthetic oestrogens from contraceptive pills and traces of many prescription medications. Germ phobia led to excessive sanitation and the overuse of antibiotics and chemical cleaning products. An increasingly indoor lifestyle developed, with less exposure to natural light during the day, and more exposure to artificial light during the night. A lack of sunlight caused widespread deficiency in vitamin D. An increasingly sedentary lifestyle set in. Stress increased, movement decreased and sleep worsened, with technology, including screens and social media, compounding these problems. The centrality of strong family and community relationships declined.

The normal balance of many hormones, including insulin, leptin, cortisol and melatonin, has been disrupted by these changes, as has the gut microbiome. As a result, rates of obesity, type 2 diabetes, chronic disease, inflammatory and allergic conditions, mental health problems and behavioural issues are all increasing in both children and adults. The very places designed to care for and nurture people, such as schools, hospitals and care homes, have become some of the worst offenders when it comes to facilitating an unhealthy lifestyle.

How well does modern healthcare do at addressing all this? How much attention is given to nutrition and lifestyle, and how much to prescribing medications and discussing side effects? Handing out medication is a quick and easy approach for a doctor who is already running late for a ten minute consultation. And it's often what patients want, since few doctors are discussing the root causes of their health issues, or coming up with sensible suggestions to address them. Billions are spent each year with this drug-based approach. The response to the increased awareness of low vitamin D levels reveals how people have been conditioned to respond to medical problems. Skin requires exposure to direct sunlight in order for the body to produce vitamin D. Rather than reversing the root cause, by getting outside in the sun more and eating whole foods high in vitamin D, which both come with additional health benefits, the focus has instead been one of using supplements for everyone, rather than just those who need them despite appropriate lifestyle changes. This of course creates the potential for profit.

There is a growing movement of people who recognise the many wrong turns that have been taken over recent decades, and who are working to help reverse these detrimental changes. Fortunately, we have the power to address many of the root causes of chronic disease without reliance on government or healthcare systems. It is down to us to make the necessary changes ourselves.

When it comes to making changes in any area of life, setting unrealistic goals is often a quick path to failure. Goals must be realistically attainable, and the rate of change must be slow in order to achieve long term success. We want to form habits and change our innate behaviour, rather than relying on high levels of self control. In the initial phase of lifestyle changes, where self control is needed, it should ideally only be required for short bursts, rather than days on end, since long periods of self control are usually not achievable. Once a new lifestyle habit has been formed, self control will no longer be required, and can be redirected towards a new goal.

To do something new consistently, it needs to be enjoyable or seen as a fun challenge, so picking changes that resonate with the user is important. Lifestyle changes often become habits more quickly if they are done every day consistently, rather than less frequently.

A slow step-by-step progression, forming a habit before moving on to the next goal, means that initial changes tend to be smaller, but longer lasting. Once an individual starts achieving their initial goals, motivation increases as they begin to feel the positive effects those changes bring. Self control is gradually needed less because of the anticipated sense of achievement that will accompany the next challenge. This causes a ripple effect, with each success impacting the next goal, aiding quicker and easier change.

It is also important to consider what the ultimate underlying goal to any lifestyle change is, since getting this right can be a make or break factor. Losing weight is, for many people, a good aspiration to have, but for it to be the only primary goal in changing nutrition and lifestyle is not always the ideal approach for success. This is because weight loss is not always easy, and for most people it takes a long time, especially if using sensible methods that yield long term results.

For this reason, it is important to have our primary focus directed towards improving our health and the way we feel (such as our energy levels), rather than weight loss. Our most fundamental goal should be to feel better, and feel good about making daily choices that improve our long term health. For those who want to lose weight, a few days of effort is not going to achieve any significant results. But if we improve our nutrition, sleep, movement or stress levels, we really can notice that we feel significantly better within just a few days, which will quickly translate into additional motivation.

Weight loss should therefore be seen as a long term outcome rather than a short term goal.

What follows are ten suggested tips for starting a journey towards a healthier, happier life. Some may sound hard, others easy. These are not supposed to be rules that must be stuck to without fail, but rather a springboard to help propel people in the right direction. Suggestions for implementing new behaviours will be given, to help turn them into long term lifestyle changes. Doing them with others, with whom you can discuss your journey, can help to make them more enjoyable.

PART 2
PRACTICAL TIPS

TIP 1: USE TIME RESTRICTED EATING

WHY? Time restricted eating, in which food consumption is limited to a certain daily time window, gives the body a long fasting period overnight which puts it into a low insulin state, reducing insulin resistance and aiding weight regulation. The gut gets sufficient rest time for repair, and prolonged time without food favours beneficial gut bacteria, some of which help in repair of the bowel wall. This can improve many gastrointestinal symptoms including bloating and IBS. This eating pattern also promotes autophagy (a clear out of old damaged cells throughout the body) which is increased in periods of fasting, as well as reducing generalised inflammation. Most people feel increased energy with time restricted eating.

Points to Consider

Time restricted eating involves eating all your food for the day within a set time window. This is sometimes referred to as intermittent fasting. A popular example of this is the 16:8 diet, which limits food intake to 8 hours each day, giving 16 hours without food in each 24 hour period. This is in contrast to the common modern eating pattern which results in the consumption of food over a period of more than 12 hours each day.

For most people, the ideal eating window will be 10 hours or less. Within the eating window, 2 or 3 meals can be eaten as normal. Snacking between meals should be avoided, since this increases the number of insulin peaks throughout the eating window. Outside the eating window, only water should be drunk, though some people also include black unsweetened tea or coffee. This means that alcohol intake is usually limited to within the context of a meal, creating more healthy drinking patterns.

Ideally, the eating window should be centred around daylight hours to optimise the gut circadian rhythm, though in winter months this may not always be practical. Avoid opening the eating window within 1 hour of waking if possible. It is important not to close the eating window late in the evening, since the time between finishing eating and bedtime is important for gut health and will impact how restorative sleep will be. It is best to close the eating window at least 2 hours before bed.

Shorter eating windows are not always better. It is not good to be in a rush to reach a deadline. Fast eating promotes overeating, since fullness hormones take time to take effect in response to food intake. Rather, slow mindful relaxed eating within a realistic eating window should be the aim. Time restricted eating does not involve calorie restriction.

Practical approach

First, consider your current eating window. If longer than 12 hours, consider this as the first goal, delaying the start of breakfast or bringing forward the end of supper, or both, in small 30-60 minute steps until you are eating within a 12 hour period. Brushing your teeth is a good way to close your eating window, and when done early can be an effective tool in helping to reduce late evening cravings.

Once a 12 hour eating window is achieved, do this regularly until it has become a habit. This will then be the baseline from which to experiment with shorter eating windows, which can be gradually implemented in incremental time steps. You may find it easy to miss breakfast in order to comfortably create a shorter eating window. If this is the case, the focus should be on avoiding closing the eating window late in the evening. If it's meal time, but you are not feeling hungry, then don't eat. We should only eat when hungry.

Time restricted eating should be fairly easy and not result in any sort of excessive hunger. If this is not the case, it will be necessary to shift the focus first to the quality of food being consumed, since overly processed foods, particularly overly processed carbohydrates, drive the desire to snack and consume food regularly over a long eating window.

TIP 2: MINIMISE OVERLY PROCESSED FOODS AND INGREDIENTS

WHY? Avoiding overly processed foods reduces the consumption of foods that contribute to glucose, fructose and insulin spikes, foods that promote inflammation and foods that are devoid of micronutrients. This avoids problems with low energy levels, malfunctioning weight regulation, insulin resistance and generalised inflammation. It also limits artificial ingredients that damage the gut microbiome. And when it comes to animal products, as well as providing better nutrition, minimising overly processed foods promotes better animal welfare. If we do not buy overly processed foods, we are voting with our wallet about the quality of food we expect to be available.

Points to Consider

The front packaging of food is designed to sell the product, not aid the consumer to make an informed decision or a healthy choice. 'Low fat' may mean high sugar. 'No added sugar' may mean artificial non-food sweeteners instead. 'Wholegrain' appears on packaging that is only partially wholegrain, and does not tell us about the overall health of the product. We should remain sceptical about messaging on food packaging that makes health claims, and instead carefully check the ingredients list ourselves, since this is the most reliable way we have of spotting overly processed foods.

It can be hard to classify exactly what counts as overly processed food, and different people have different opinions. We have found applying the following five checks when looking at the ingredients list works well for identifying what might be considered overly processed foods:

1. Any sugar or sweetening product
2. Any grain unless 100% wholegrain
3. Any oil unless it is virgin or extra virgin
4. Any non-food ingredients
5. Intensively farmed meat, fish and animal products

Foods that contain any of the items in this five point checklist would be classified as overly processed. Let us consider these categories further.

1. Any sugar or sweetening product

This includes sugar, sucrose, glucose, fructose, corn syrup, cane juice, maltose, dextrose, fruit juice concentrate, and artificial sweeteners such as sucralose and aspartame. We should remain suspicious of all sweetening products appearing on the label even when they claim to be from fruit. Even honey, when used as an added ingredient, is likely to be poor quality and is best avoided. It will always be best to add sweetening products ourselves at home, ideally by using just whole fruit. Agave syrup is a classic example of a sweetener being promoted as good because it has a lower GI than other sweeteners due to its lower glucose content. However, this is because it has a much higher fructose content, which is not a good trade off.

2. Any grain unless 100% wholegrain

This means any wheat, rice, oats, corn or other grain, in products such as bread, pasta and cereals, that is not 100% wholegrain (sometimes referred to as wholemeal when milled into flour, or wholewheat in reference to wheat). Beware that in many products labelled wholegrain, when checking the ingredients list the first ingredient may indeed be a wholegrain, such as 'wholegrain wheat', but the next ingredient may simply be 'wheat', meaning that it is not wholegrain. This means the product contains overly processed grains, and is only partially wholegrain. Regarding sourdough breads, a true sourdough will not have yeast appearing on the ingredients list, though breads marketed as sourdough often have yeast listed, meaning that a bit of sourdough has been added as a token gesture to an otherwise standard packet yeast risen loaf.

3. Any oil unless it is virgin or extra virgin

Virgin refers to oil that has been extracted by basic mechanical means only, rather than using high heat, solvents or chemical processes. The aim here is to eliminate all highly processed seed oils, as well as highly processed palm oil and overly processed olive oils or deodorised coconut oils. Instead, the only oils consumed should be high quality minimally processed fruit oils such as extra virgin olive oil, virgin avocado oil and virgin coconut oil. Beware that regulations surrounding the use of terms like virgin vary significantly between different countries, and so it is best to check that the oil is cold pressed without any chemical processing or deodorising if you are unsure. You can now find virgin seed oils such as virgin rapeseed oil. However, as previously stated, these seed oils contain high percentages of polyunsaturated fat and so are inherently unstable once produced and stored, and even more so when cooked with. They still represent a new addition to the human diet, putting the regular user into a human experiment on the long term health effects. Extra virgin olive oil has been used for thousands of years and, as a hallmark of the Mediterranean diet, is a much safer bet. Again, beware of labelling trickery, with one example being hummus advertised as being made with extra virgin olive oil despite having seed oil higher up on the ingredients list.

4. Any non-food ingredients

This includes E numbers, preservatives, artificial sweeteners, nitrites, emulsifiers, or any other ingredient that you could not buy yourself. If you wouldn't keep it in your kitchen to add to your own cooking, then avoid food containing it.

5. Intensively farmed meat, fish and animal products

This includes all farmed fish. Fish should be wild only, and the label should tell you where it was caught and with what fishing method. If unclear, it can be assumed to have been intensively farmed. Meat, dairy and eggs should be from wild or pasture raised animals that graze outside on their natural diet (such as grass) as much as possible. If this is not clear on the package, then we can assume a poor quality product. These things should be checked when buying fresh at the counter too. Meat and animal products contained within other products, such as in ready meals or in pre-made sandwiches or pizzas, are almost always going to be poor quality.

Where possible, it is always best to aim for organic food grown without the use of harmful pesticides and chemical fertilisers, that damage both the environment and the consumer. Plants grown in more healthy organic soils will tend to have more micronutrients. An exception to the rule would be fish labelled as organic, since organic fish is by definition farmed because a wild animal cannot be classified in this manner. More generally, just because something is organic does not mean it is not overly processed, so organic products that contain overly processed ingredients should also be minimised, though they are certainly a lot better than their non-organic counterparts. Once again, different countries have significant variations in the regulation of what farming standards can be classed as organic or not. Engaging with small suppliers to buy local produce can help to provide more clarity and often a superior product.

The nutritional information labelling given on food packets does not indicate how processed a food is, and so rarely provides useful information as to how healthy a food is. Calorie labelling is often inaccurate and does not take into account that not all the calories in food will be absorbed into the bloodstream, especially in the case of whole foods due to their more complex food matrix. Calorie content does not help determine the way a food will impact health or long term weight, since it gives no indication of the quality of the food or how processed it is. The quality of calories consumed is far more important than the quantity, since it is the action food has on hormone systems and internal physiology that determines good health and weight regulation. The same amount of calories can have vastly different effects on the body, depending on the type and quality of the food consumed.

Those wishing to have low salt intake may wish to check salt content on the nutritional information label. Overly processed foods often have a high salt content. In the context of an unprocessed diet and healthy lifestyle, regulating salt intake is usually not necessary. Similarly, the carbohydrate/fibre ratio, protein content and fat content can all be checked for interest's sake if wanted. The amount of fat and protein in food is not a useful indicator of how healthy or how processed it is. This includes the breakdown of fat types. Most people instinctively know which foods are high in fat and high in protein, and both will be beneficial to include in meals. Both are essential macronutrients that are effective at signalling fullness, whilst also helping to dampen the insulin response to the carbohydrate portion of a meal.

Practical approach

An initial goal of never eating overly processed foods again would of course be a very unrealistic starting point. The goal here is to minimise, not necessarily completely eliminate, overly processed foods. This is an ongoing task, and small changes should be made in incremental steps, levelling out at a point that can be maintained easily in the long term. Start by looking through the foods you have at home, becoming familiar with spotting overly processed ingredients, and considering the sort of foods that contain these ingredients.

An initial goal could then be to eliminate any drinks with overly processed ingredients. This would mean avoiding any sweet or sugary drinks, including tea or coffee with added sugar. Although fruit juices may not fit in the overly processed categories above, much of the fibre in the fruit that the juice came from has been removed, and what is left is a drink that can cause a very large insulin response and deliver a high fructose load. We also want to train our taste buds away from regular consumption of sweet things. Therefore all sweetened drinks, including juices, are best avoided. The next goal could then be to avoid snacks that are overly processed.

Snacks are best avoided altogether, but if having one, stick to something unprocessed, savoury, and simple such as a boiled egg or unsalted nuts. Both sweet drinks and regular snacking on overly processed foods are big drivers in childhood obesity and behavioural issues, so this is an important step for children to take as well as adults.

Once avoiding overly processed drinks and snacks has become a habit, move on to tackling meals, one meal at a time. Start by aiming to have the first meal of the day without any overly processed foods or ingredients. Once you have established this as a habit, you can explore moving onto other meals of the day. The more you become aware of overly processed foods and get into the habit of checking ingredients labelling for them, the more you will find yourself naturally wanting to avoid them, without the need for high levels of self control.

When you get a craving for some overly processed foods, say a sweet drink or some chocolate, try to include it with a meal. Consuming overly processed foods in the context of an otherwise healthy balanced meal will have much less of a problematic effect on your body compared to when consumed alone. It is also likely you'll eat less overly processed food when eaten after a main course rather than on an empty stomach. Foods with sugar in will cause a much more significant insulin response when eaten in isolation, compared with being consumed after a meal containing fibre, protein and fat. This is a good time to utilise short term self control. Put the chocolate to one side, telling yourself you can have it after the main course of your next meal. You might find that after eating, you no longer feel the need for it, but if you do, enjoy it as a reward for delaying its consumption.

Using the same principle, the insulin response to any meal can be altered by changing the eating order of foods on the plate. By eating fibre rich foods first, and carbohydrate dominant foods last, the glucose absorption rate will be slowed and the insulin rise blunted. Vinegar is another food known to reduce glucose and insulin spikes by slowing digestion and absorption of carbohydrates, and it also directly improves insulin sensitivity. As an example, eating bread for lunch after having consumed a salad dressed with vinegar will have a significant effect on how the body responds to the carbohydrates in the bread.

Drinking herbal tea to finish a meal can be a helpful way to diffuse cravings for overly processed sweet foods. Being adequately hydrated throughout the day will also help. Getting rid of tempting overly processed foods from the house helpfully limits availability. Avoid going shopping when hungry to reduce the temptation to stock up on these foods in the first place.

The most important factor when it comes to this tip is to start with simple steps and progress gradually, since we want to create long lasting changes, rather than a short term diet. Level off at a sustainable place for you, since further progress can always be made in the future.

TIP 3: MAXIMISE THE VARIETY OF HEALTHY FOOD

WHY? Maximising food variety helps support the diversity of beneficial bacteria in the gut microbiome. It also ensures that all the essential fats and proteins that the body requires are consumed, along with a good range of different micronutrients needed for general health and weight regulation. Having a wide variety of flavours helps retrain taste buds away from the monotony of overly processed foods.

Points to Consider

The following are some examples of unprocessed or minimally processed foods that can be included in a varied diet:

> **1. Vegetables:** green vegetables (e.g. asparagus, broad beans, broccoli, brussel sprouts, cabbage, cavolo nero, celery, chinese leaf, courgette, cucumber, fennel, garden peas, green beans, kale, leek, lettuce, mange tout, pak choi, rocket, runner beans, samphire, seaweed, spinach, spring onion, sprouting seed, sugar snap peas, swiss chard, watercress) and colourful vegetables (e.g. artichoke, aubergine, cauliflower, chicory, garlic, mushrooms, pepper, purple onion, radish, red cabbage, rhubarb, shallots, tomatoes).

2. Carbohydrates: ground or root vegetables (e.g beetroot, carrot, celeriac, parsnip, potato, pumpkin, squash, swede, sweet potato, turnip), legumes (e.g black beans, butter beans, cannellini beans, chickpeas, kidney beans, lentils, pinto beans, split peas), and wholegrains (e.g. amaranth, barley, buckwheat, einkorn, emmer, kamut, maize, oat, quinoa, rice, rye, spelt).

3. Proteins: eggs, milk, cheese, meat (including the muscle, fat, offal and bone broth of animals e.g beef, buffalo, chicken, duck, lamb, goat, partridge, pheasant, pigeon, quail, turkey, venison), and fish (e.g anchovies, bass, bream, cod, haddock, hake, halibut, herring, mackerel, plaice, pollock, wild salmon, sardines, sole, tilapia, trout, tuna).

4. Fats: extra virgin olive oil, butter, cream, olives, cacao nibs, avocado, coconut, nuts (e.g. almonds, brazil nuts, cashews, chestnuts, hazelnuts, macadamias, peanuts, pecans, pinenuts, pistachios, walnuts), and seeds (e.g. chia, flax, hemp, poppy, pumpkin, sesame, squash, sunflower).

5. Fermented foods: cheese (preferably made with unpasteurised/raw milk e.g. camembert, cheddar, comte, emmental, gruyere, manchego, parmesan, roquefort), live yoghurt including kefir, sourdough bread, kimchi, sauerkraut, fermented pickles, fermented pico de gallo, vinegar (e.g balsamic, raw apple cider, red wine, sherry), miso, tamari, kombucha, red wine, tea and coffee.

6. Herbs, herbal teas and spices: allspice, aniseed, basil, bay, black pepper, capers, cardamom, carraway, cayenne, chamomile, chervil, chilli, chives. cinnamon, clove, coriander, cumin, curry, dandelion, dill, echinacea, elderflower, eucalyptus, fennel seed, fenugreek, ginger, hibiscus, juniper, lavender, lemon balm, licorice, maca, marjoram, matcha, mint, mustard, nettle, nutmeg, oregano, paprika, parsley, peppermint, pine needle, raspberry leaf, rose hip, rosemary, saffron, sage, star anise, sumac, swedish bitters, tarragon, thai basil, thyme, turmeric, vanilla, and za'atar.

7. Fruits: such as apple, apricot, banana, baobab, bilberry, blackberry, blackcurrant, blueberry, cherry, clementine, cranberry, date, fig, goji berry, gooseberry, grapefruit (grapefruit can alter the blood concentration of certain drugs, so this should be checked if you are on medication), grapes, kiwi, lemon, lime, loganberry, lychee, mango, melon, mulberry, nectarine, orange, papaya, passionfruit, peach, pear, physalis, plum, pomegranate, raspberry and redcurrant.

Many of these categories overlap, and so these divisions are not set in stone. In the context of a diverse meal, proportions of macronutrients on the plate are not something that need to be strictly regulated or remain constant from meal to meal. But it is worth bearing in mind the common approach that has clearly not worked at a population level. The classic food plate or food pyramid usually has starchy carbohydrates, particularly grains, as the biggest portion. This has often led to people consuming wheat two or three times a day, with food such as pasta or bread, often overly processed, making up half or more of the plate each time. Combined with a focus on low fat, this has led to unbalanced meals which produce large insulin responses. As an example, breakfast cereal with a reduced fat milk followed by toast and washed down with orange juice is likely to give a high insulin start to the day with poor macronutrient variety. Maximising variety will help prevent basing nutrition on a single food.

Some food plates now show half the plate containing green and colourful vegetables, and the other half divided between protein, carbohydrate and fat. As a rough guide, this is probably a safe bet for most people. However, the ideal food plate is not a fixed target and will vary from person to person depending on starting point, long term goals, and other factors including levels of physical activity, personal preferences (such as if following a low carbohydrate eating pattern), culture, and the time of year if eating seasonally. The quality of food consumed should always remain the priority.

Practical approach

It can be fun to explore new and different foods which will help maximise variety. Engage a spirit of adventure to explore new tastes. Experimenting with fermented food is a good way of consuming healthy foods. Sauerkraut and kefir are examples of fermented foods that are cheap and easy to make yourself at home. Where possible, select local organic in-season produce. Try engaging your family in the process and discuss what to buy and cook together. Growing herbs in a window box or fruit and vegetables in the garden is another good way to engage with healthy eating and living. Avoid peeling root vegetables, since the skin is where much of the fibre and micronutrients are.

Reducing the need for sweet food is an important step towards better health. If you have a craving for something more sweet than fruit with your pudding, pick a locally produced cold extracted and unpasteurised (raw) honey and use in small amounts. Good quality honey provides micronutrients and adding it yourself will give an awareness of how much is being used. If you want chocolate after a meal, try experimenting with darker and darker chocolate, eating it slowly and mindfully in order to enjoy the more satisfying bittersweet taste. As your taste buds get used to the flavours of a minimally processed diet, you will find craving for sweet chocolate disappearing.

Alcohol and caffeine can be consumed in moderation, and it is best to have both alcohol and caffeine free days during the week. Consider that both, especially in excess, can exacerbate or even cause some health problems. For example, both caffeine and alcohol can cause bladder muscle instability leading to the need to pass urine more frequently, including at night, and a sudden urgency when the need arises. Caffeine and alcohol commonly cause or worsen irritation of the stomach lining (gastritis) and acid reflux.

People can be quick to reach for drugs rather than trialling exclusion periods. As with using time restricted eating and elimination of overly processed foods, we should be quick to trial lifestyle interventions such as reduction or elimination of alcohol and/or caffeine, rather than heading straight for medication. If these interventions don't work, they will have been done without risk, whilst also giving insight into the role of alcohol or caffeine in your life.

Many people feel they have a problem with grains (particularly wheat) or dairy. Often, simply a change in the quality of these foods, along with a reduction to a more moderate intake, will improve symptoms, especially when combined with time restricted eating.

The pesticide glyphosate is used on many grains for pre-harvest desiccation, where it's role is to kill the crop and make harvesting more efficient. This means many cereals and grain products that are non-organic have high levels of glyphosate that can severely impact the consumer's gut microbiome, and so switching to organic is always a wise choice. Doing this as well as trying other grains such as wholegrain rye, and picking sourdough where able, makes for a good bread choice. Wholegrain rye bread comes with the additional benefit of having a fibre proportion around three times higher than many wholegrain wheat loaves.

For those who feel dairy causes a problem, once again quality of product can make all the difference. Some people report better digestion with unpasterised (raw) milk than with pasterised milk. This may be due to the presence of higher levels of beneficial bacteria and enzymes in unpasterised milk, or that those sourcing raw milk tend to get it from animals raised to a higher standard, which gives a better quality product. Some people find symptoms related to dairy consumption resolve when they switch to goats milk, sheep's milk or A2 cow's milk (milk high in the A2 milk protein). As always, the quality of food consumed should remain the priority. It may also be worth exploring if it is dairy as a whole causing an issue, or just lactose. This can be determined by eliminating dairy with the exception of fully fermented cheese without any lactose (check the nutritional label to make sure it contains 0.1g or less of carbohydrates per 100 grams). If this is well tolerated, it may just be lactose causing a problem, in which case sticking to fermented dairy may eliminate any issues.

Some examples of meal options include:

1. Breakfast bowl containing preferred combination of kefir / mixed nuts / chia seeds / flax seeds / hemp / cacao nibs / oats, topped with fruit and flavoured with ginger / maca / nutmeg / cinnamon / vanilla.

2. Fried eggs / omelette, purple onion and spinach, with sauerkraut / kimchi / fermented pico de gallo, and rye bread toast.

3. Salad with lettuce / watercress / chicory / rocket, plus tomatoes / pepper / cucumber / avocado / spring onion / red onion, topped with pumpkin / sesame seeds. Add hard boiled eggs / fish / cheese, and herbs such as mint / parsley / coriander / basil / za'atar. Dress with extra virgin olive oil and vinegar.

4. Oven roasted chopped vegetable combination such as aubergine / courgette / onion / garlic / leek / tomatoes / pepper cooked in extra virgin olive oil, with rosemary / chilli / other herbs or spices, along with roasted root vegetable mix on a separate tray, plus fried or baked fish / meat of choice.

5. Pasta based meals, such as spaghetti bolognese, but with the pasta replaced with cougettini / black beans / lentils / cauliflower, and with plenty of different vegetables cut up in the sauce, topped with cheese.

6. Roast dinner with lamb / pheasant and roasted vegetables such as potatoes / beetroot / parsnips / shallots / garlic / fennel / cabbage wedges.

7. Oxtail soup with celery, carrot, onion and red wine, which can be cooked on the stove / in a slow cooker / in a pressure cooker. Heart / liver can also be added. Served with barley/quinoa.

8. Steak and kidney pie with onions, mushrooms, swede and homemade bone broth. Add basic pie crust or cook as a stew, with a side of green beans / swiss chard.

9. Curry made using coconut milk and preferred spice combination / curry powder, with cod / chicken / chickpeas, and pak choi / broccoli / roasted brussel sprouts.

10. Simple pudding options include the breakfast bowl above, fruit salad, a cheese board, and herbal tea. There are now many alternative pudding recipes such as chocolate avocado mousse (blended avocado, cacao powder and honey, flavoured with vanilla extract / lime juice), and kidney bean chocolate cake (using kidney beans, cacao powder, dates, eggs and coconut oil).

Healthy foods should be delicious and enjoyable. By having a wide-ranging diet, you get to spend less time thinking about specific micronutrients or the breakdown of macronutrients, and more time exploring different cuisines.

TIP 4: MAXIMISE OUTDOOR MORNING LIGHT

WHY? Early morning exposure to natural outdoor light sets the master clock for the day. It eliminates any remaining melatonin and aids the beneficial morning peak in cortisol, helping normalise cortisol circadian rhythm. Getting outside first thing provides full alertness without reliance on caffeine. Exposure to bright outdoor natural light is also important for reducing the risk of short-sightedness, an increasingly common problem due to indoor lifestyles. Getting outside in the mornings improves mental health, increases energy levels, and boosts morning focus and attention levels.

Points to Consider

The aim here is to get outside into natural light as soon as possible after waking, ideally before breakfast, and to maximise time outdoors throughout the morning.

We want plenty of time spent outdoors in natural bright light throughout the day, though the morning is particularly useful for setting healthy circadian rhythms and is often under prioritised in the morning rush. Sun glasses will dampen the effectiveness of the bright light, so avoid wearing them in the morning unless absolutely necessary.

Practical approach

It can sometimes be hard to want to get out first thing in the morning, but doing so will bring with it an instant improvement in alertness. Going in the garden for a short time or taking just a brief stroll up and down the block will have a big impact. Getting out early is also great to do with others, including children, even if just for a few minutes.

During winter months, if it is dark on waking, getting out will still certainly help wake you up, though a priority should be placed on getting outside as soon as it is light. If commuting to work, this may mean leaving ten minutes earlier so that upon arriving, you can take a stroll outside before starting work. Go outside in any breaks that you have.

Time in the morning is often limited, but this is sometimes due to sleeping in late and struggling to wake up. This is a result of insufficient amounts of good quality sleep, and being out in the morning light begins the process towards better sleep the following night. Relying on caffeine to make us fully alert is a symptom of insufficient good quality sleep, or dependence on caffeine, or both. In these cases, it is best to consider a caffeine detox for a week, followed by reintroduction at a more moderate level, with caffeine free days incorporated to avoid future dependence.

Aim to consume caffeinated drinks only once fully awake, ideally after having already been outside. The rationale for this is due to caffeine's mechanism of action. Caffeine is thought to increase alertness by blocking adenosine, a neurotransmitter in the brain that causes tiredness. Morning activity such as moving outside in natural light reduces adenosine levels, whereas blocking adenosine before levels have reduced allows it to persist. Once the caffeine begins to wear off, tiredness can therefore return, contributing to a slump in energy in the afternoon.

> The ease at which this tip is able to be followed is of course in part determined by what you do the night before.

TIP 5: MINIMISE ARTIFICIAL LIGHTING AND SCREENS AFTER 8PM

WHY? Darkness drives melatonin production and helps promote good quality sleep, which is important for reducing inflammation and improving insulin sensitivity. In addition to the disrupting effects of the light emitted, avoiding screens stops exposure to stimulating or stress inducing activities in the evening such as looking at the news, scrolling social media or watching TV. Avoiding screens also frees up time to allow more meaningful evening activities. Minimising bright or overly stimulating environments after dark prompts an earlier bedtime giving the opportunity for longer sleep, since people naturally feel ready for bed earlier without these artificial circadian rhythm disruptors. This contributes to feeling refreshed and energised on waking, which is crucial for making healthy choices throughout the rest of the day. Waking earlier frees up more time in the morning, giving a less stressful start to the day.

Points to Consider

After dark, where practically possible, it is beneficial to limit bright overhead artificial lighting and minimise the use of screens including TV, computer and phone. 8pm is an arbitrary cut off that we have chosen. Ideally, seasonal rhythms would be followed, with bright light and screen exposure limited to daylight hours. If you can adjust and minimise artificial lighting and screens earlier in the winter months, this will be very beneficial. However, depending on where you live and the time of year, this may be completely impractical. We feel 8pm is a good compromise as general guidance, though this can be personalised to your needs. In summer, even if it remains bright outside past 8pm, avoiding screens after this time will still promote more wholesome activities rather than sitting and watching TV.

Unlike screens and bright overhead lighting, fire does not disrupt melatonin production or our body clocks. This is because it gives off low light levels at the low energy red coloured end of the light spectrum. If lights are needed after your cut off time, try to keep to those that most resemble fire (dim, low down, amber tones) rather than those that resemble daytime sun (bright, overhead, white).

Practical approach

If 8pm sounds far too early for you, aim to start 30 mins before what you consider a sensible bedtime. As you learn what you enjoy filling this time with, it will become easier to shift the start time further away from your planned bedtime. As you do, you may notice that you feel ready for bed earlier and that your bedtime naturally creeps forward, which indicates that the changes being made are effective. Continue moving the cut off time earlier and earlier until you reach a point that you can realistically sustain as an ongoing lifestyle. Of course if you can move it earlier than 8pm, the benefits will keep increasing.

To prepare for this cut off, it is best to do any pre-bedtime activity that requires light, such as cleaning your teeth or setting an alarm, early in the evening. This means when you are tired and ready for sleep, you can simply get straight into bed without turning lights on or looking at your phone. Doing these activities at or shortly after the closure of your eating window is a useful habit to get into. At cut off time, phones can be put on flight mode and wifi turned off. If you think of things you need to do the following day as you get into bed, and tend to write them on your phone, have a pen and paper by the bed to use instead. This can also be a useful exercise for jotting down any thoughts that might be playing on your mind.

Plan what you are going to do after your cut off time. If doing it on your own, you may decide to go for a relaxing evening stroll, star gaze, read a book, do some stretching whilst listening to music, relax by a fire, do a puzzle, or listen to an audiobook. If doing it with family, plan activities you will do together, which can include all of the above, as well as planned time to chat with your spouse, telling stories to your children, or family activities such as a board game. This time could provide the opportunity to make a big difference in building close family relationships and reducing stress.

TIP 6: DO A 2 MINUTE BREATHING EXERCISE EACH DAY

WHY? Breathing exercises dampen any fight-or-flight response and return the body to rest-and-digest mode, helping restore a healthy autonomic nervous system balance and contributing to the normalisation of cortisol. They help train the body to breathe in and out through the nose using the diaphragm. The more slow nasal breathing exercises are practised consciously, the more they will also happen subconsciously, including when asleep. This can reduce blood pressure, stress and tension, improve mental health and digestion, and help decrease generalised inflammation and insulin resistance caused by raised cortisol.

Points to Consider

There are many different breathing exercises that all involve slow conscious breathing. One example would be slowly breathing in for a count of five, then slowly out for a count of 5, followed by a pause, and then continuing this pattern for 2 minutes. Another option is box breathing, which involves breathing in for a count of 4, pausing for a count of 4, breathing out for a count of 4, then pausing again for a count of 4, and continuing this pattern for 2 minutes.

Practical approach

Pick a time and place that will give you a comfortable and relaxed environment to do these exercises. If you haven't had a chance earlier in the day, they can be done in bed to help relax and promote sleep. Start by considering how you are breathing, whether you are using your chest or belly, and if breathing through your mouth or nose. Simply becoming consciously aware of your breath will tend to slow the breathing rate. Then begin your preferred pattern, using your belly to breathe in and out through your nose.

Once practised, you may want to insert these exercises at various points in your day. They can be done before meals to improve digestion. They can also be used as a tool in stressful situations, such as in a work meeting or before a job interview, to help improve performance. You will find yourself becoming more aware of your breathing as you go about your day, and this will help reinforce the pattern.

TIP 7: DO A 1 MINUTE MINDSET EXERCISE EACH DAY

WHY? Mindset exercises help to reframe perspective towards one of positivity, gratitude, optimism, and growth. This can help reduce stress and improve mental health, helping rebalance the autonomic nervous system and normalise cortisol, contributing to a more enjoyable day.

Points to Consider

A mindset exercise could be any activity that helps you slow down and consciously improve your frame of mind. It is usually best done in the morning, to help set your outlook for the day. However, mindset exercises may be used effectively at any point. This could be a deliberate activity such as prayer, meditation, mindfulness, journaling, taking time to consider what you are grateful for, telling someone in your family what you appreciate about them, or using positive affirmations to remind yourself of your own good traits and challenge excessive self criticism. It could also be setting time aside to do an activity that you know improves your mindset, such as putting on uplifting music, playing a musical instrument, dancing, walking outside in your garden barefoot to feel a connection to the ground, reading an inspiring book or poetry, or listening to an encouraging podcast.

The idea here is not to deny the hardships of life or any difficulties you may be going through. Similarly, we are not trying to numb ourselves from natural times of sadness and grief, the suppression of which would be bad for both mental and physical health. It is certainly important to acknowledge and consider these sorts of issues, embracing them as part of normal life. Rather, the idea is to balance the mind with a healthy amount of positivity, which should then allow us to become more open and honest about hard situations we find ourselves in, whilst simultaneously helping to stop them from dominating our lives. In an ideal situation, these sorts of mindset activities should be part of our innate behaviour rather than exercises that need practising. However, in our modern societies, due to the prevalence of unhealthy thought patterns, for many people it has become increasingly essential to foster and develop a calmer, more positive mindset as a stepping stone towards better health.

Practical Approach:

Consider what activity appeals to you, what you feel you can keep up on a regular basis and what time of day will be best to make it habitual. Since this is the sort of activity that often becomes a low priority during a busy day, time doing it can be kept short, and it may be necessary to set an alarm as a prompt.

As with any of the tips given, if it sounds unappealing or you have little motivation to do it, do not force yourself, since long lasting lifestyle changes will not be successful with this approach. Instead focus on changes that appeal, revisiting other ones later when you feel motivated and ready.

TIP 8: USE THE ONE-IN, ONE-OUT RULE OF MINIMALISM

WHY? Embracing some degree of minimalism, a way of living with the minimal amount of required possessions, can help people break free from the culture of materialism and consumerism. It also helps reduce clutter. For many people, clutter adds more stress to life. A decluttered house saves time with cleaning and tidying, and often leads to a decluttered mind. Minimalism also makes us more mindful of what we actually need, rather than buying unnecessary stuff that is quickly thrown away. This all helps to save money, free up time, and reduce the environmental impact of excessive turnover, particularly of things made of plastic. Minimalism helps us refocus our sense of pleasure and satisfaction, so that we can derive it from meaningful activities and relationships rather than material goods.

Points to Consider

The one-in, one-out method is a good way to begin minimalism. Each time you bring a new item into your possession, get rid of something you already have. The idea here is not to promote a high turnover of possessions, but rather to help reduce the accumulation of more and more stuff, and to help us become more mindful of what we spend our money on. This applies equally to children, whose imagination is often not exercised fully due to the presence of excess toy clutter along with ever increasing screen time, causing endless distraction and an erosion of the creative spirit that imagination helps nurture. We want to change our mindset from that of consumerism that wants us to ask 'what more do I need?', and instead ask ourselves 'do I have enough?'

Practical Approach

A good way to start this is with a thorough declutter of your property and possessions. Hold onto those things that improve physical or mental health, or enhance relationships by encouraging shared activity. With everything else, carefully consider whether they are really needed and if not sell them or take them to a charity shop. If you live with others, try to involve them in this process. This includes children, with whom you can discuss which items are enjoyable and productive and which are just causing clutter and mess. This may prompt a discussion on the importance of not deriving happiness from unnecessary material possessions.

Once this new decluttered baseline has been established, start the one-in, one-out rule. We naturally do this with food, buying new food once we have used the old and need more. The same can be applied on most occasions for any other category you spend money on, from electronic items to clothes to children's toys.

This rule can still be applied at birthdays and holidays such as Christmas. These events have often come to be dominated by consumerism and materialism, leading to an excess of accumulated junk, often plastic, much of which quickly ends up in landfill. Celebrations may cause people financial stress due to the excess spending that they feel duty bound to make.

If needed, explain to friends, relatives, or children that your gifts may be non-material. This might include a gift to bring a home cooked meal round to a relatives house, or taking your children camping or on a trip to a local farm. If you want to give physical gifts, for adults you could consider healthy foods, such as a premium bottle of organic extra virgin olive oil or a hamper including organic 100% grass fed beef, or other foods that you think would be appreciated. For children, stick to things that you would buy them even if it wasn't a birthday, such as buying your child a new bike if they have outgrown their last one. You can also ask others to reciprocate, freeing them from felt obligation, whilst opening up a discussion about your reasoning. The time and money saved can be fed into making these special occasions stand out in more meaningful ways, and may well improve relationships.

> Minimalism and decluttering tend to be both psychologically satisfying and contagious. Making simple changes will often inspire others to follow suit.

TIP 9: MOVE EVERY 30 MINS

WHY? Moving frequently throughout the day improves insulin sensitivity, helps normalise cortisol and combat stress, and improves sleep. It also helps reduce musculoskeletal pains and a wide range of chronic diseases associated with a sedentary lifestyle, which include many cancers. It increases energy levels and concentration.

Points to Consider

We want to move as much as possible throughout the day. Most of this movement represents non-exercise activity, though most days should ideally include some exercise as well, with a combination of strength and endurance exercise undertaken during each week. Non-exercise activity undertaken after a meal has a useful impact on reducing the insulin response to a meal, and so avoiding insulin resistance. Moving and exercising outside in nature comes with additional benefits including exposure to bright outdoor light, the potential for vitamin D synthesis, and an environment conducive to improving mental health and benefiting the gut microbiome.

Practical approach

Starting early, with movement outside first thing in the morning is a good pattern to set if you are able. Aim to walk, rather than drive, where possible. If doing sedentary work, try setting a repeating timer for every 30 mins to prompt movement. At these 30 minute intervals, a minute can be taken to walk up and down the stairs, take a break outside, or do some brief exercise such as squats, lunges, press ups or star jumps. This pattern can be continued into the evening, including if watching TV where it will help break up screen time. In all situations, it really is a case of the more movement and the less time sitting in chairs, the better. Actively look for opportunities to move more, such as taking the stairs rather than a lift, walking or biking rather than driving, or playing at the playground with your children or grandchildren rather than sitting and watching. You could get a standing desk to help vary the number of stationary positions you adopt, or even consider a walking treadmill to go under the standing desk.

When it comes to exercise, pick a mix of activities during the week which could include power walking, running, strength training, cycling, swimming, sports, dancing, yoga, pilates, aerobics or any other type of activity that you fancy. Strength training can be done using body weight exercises, resistance bands, or weights. Remember to include activities that target core muscle groups (including the glutes) in your chosen weekly activities. If pushed for time, just 5-10 minutes of high intensity interval training is a good choice that comes with its own unique benefits. Intense physical exercise should ideally be avoided in the evening since it can cause a spike in cortisol and delay evening relaxation and sleep.

When choosing footwear, we can avoid future generations from having to suffer the problems associated with modern shoes by encouraging our children to be barefoot as much as possible, and buying them minimalist shoes, which provide warmth and protection only. Proper minimalist footwear should have a wide toe box allowing the toes to splay out whilst walking, but have no cushioning, no support, and no heel rise. Providing children with this sort of footwear will allow their walking and running patterns to develop naturally. Adults considering transitioning to minimalist footwear should do so gradually and carefully, starting with walking, not running, whilst incorporating foot strengthening exercises and foot stretches, with advice from someone who understands the process. It may be that foot changes that have already occurred in the feet due to years of modern footwear make the transition problematic and so care is advised, although in almost all cases avoiding footwear with a narrow toe box or significant heel rise will be beneficial.

We should be encouraging children to move as much as possible throughout the day. We should also encourage them to sit on the floor without support rather than on chairs when sitting is required, since this will help them retain their natural mobility and core strength. For adults, sitting on the floor in a variety of proper ground sitting positions whilst watching TV instead of sitting on a sofa will naturally encourage fidgeting and regular changes in position. This may also encourage our bodies to recover some of the lost mobility that comes from excessive time in chairs.

Mirroring natural movement patterns as much as possible, especially when done outside in nature, will help both our physical and mental health.

TIP 10: DO ONE ACTIVITY EACH WEEK THAT IS BOTH A PHYSICAL AND MENTAL CHALLENGE

WHY? Having a challenge of this nature helps improve resilience to other types of stress you may encounter, whilst also giving a sense of accomplishment when achieved. These hormetic stressors train the body to move efficiently out of a fight-or-flight response. Many of them also come with additional health benefits. For example, fasting promotes autophagy, reduces inflammation and improves insulin sensitivity. Cold water exposure increases insulin sensitivity, decreases blood pressure, improves immunity and elevates mood. These activities also serve to develop a spirit of adventure for new challenges, which is a useful approach to help drive change through exploring new lifestyle measures.

Points to Consider

Examples that could be chosen include fasting for 20-24 hours, taking a cold shower, cold water swimming, a hard physical exercise challenge, a hormetic breathing challenge such as cyclic hyperventilation (e.g. Wim Hof breathing), going for a long walk in the rain, or any other challenge that appeals.

By definition, any sort of hormetic stress or challenge is dose dependent. This means that having the right amount results in benefit, but overdoing it can do more harm than good. An example with exercise would be overtraining, where fatigue, injury and chronic inflammation can set in. The thresholds for this will be different for everyone, but can be gauged by how you feel overall upon completion of the activity and in the long run.

Practical approach

These challenges will often be more fun if done with others where possible. Doing challenges with others also means you can spur each other on and celebrate success afterwards. Pick something that appeals and plan a good time to do it. It could be the same activity each week or something different.

Don't worry if you set a challenge and then fall short of your initial expectations. You will still have challenged yourself and may be motivated to revisit the challenge another week after considering any additional steps that could be taken to help achieve that goal. Above all, these challenges should be enjoyable, so if you do not look forward to one, switch to another.

CONCLUSION

Chronic disease and obesity are an expression of our bodies no longer being able to cope with, or compensate for, modern living. Modern medicine is unable to address or resolve the root causes that drive the problem. Lifestyle changes that improve health simply act to challenge these unhealthy patterns of modern living, in order to break free from the consequences.

At their core, no lifestyle interventions are complicated. They involve basic things such as being conscious of proper breathing, eating real food, minimising exposure to chemicals, using medication only when absolutely necessary and for as short a time as possible, getting outside into nature, moving frequently, avoiding late night screens, getting good sleep, and cultivating family and community life. All things we instinctively know to be beneficial.

All age groups, including children, need good nutrition and lifestyle habits in order to thrive. There is no reason to wait for problems to set in before addressing these factors. We should be training the next generation for a healthy future, with the examples we set now helping to determine this. We can also learn a lot about healthy lifestyles from young children. They are constantly moving and cannot sit still, yet hate to be in a rush, enjoy taking their time at meals, and get pleasure from simple things such as playing together, getting outside into nature, or reading a book with family. They have a growth mindset, are adaptable and positive, and are always looking for opportunities to explore and learn. Modern patterns of living are causing these traits to disappear at an increasingly early age, but once we recognise this we can help to nurture these characteristics and prevent them from being eroded.

Each day brings with it choices that can improve health or worsen it. The food and lifestyle choices we make can promote health or promote disease. Our actions will influence those around us. The way we spend our money will influence what sort of products businesses sell us. These are our votes for the future that count the most. We all need to take personal responsibility and unprocess our lives as much as possible. This will bring us increased energy to enjoy a more happy, healthy, and meaningful life.

WHAT'S NEXT?

We created Bosanquet Health in order to help people take steps towards improving their health and happiness. Our company provides education and support with personalised nutrition and lifestyle plans. Our range of services include private consultations, group courses, talks, and bespoke packages for clients with specific goals.

You can email us at BosanquetHealth@gmail.com or find out more on our website BosanquetHealth.com where you can sign up to receive updates and regular free health tips.

BIBLIOGRAPHY

Bikman, B. (2021). *Why We Get Sick*. Dallas, TX: BenBella Books.

Chatterjee, R. (2018). *The Stress Solution*. London, UK: Penguin Life.

Foster, R. G. (2022). *Life Time*. London, UK: Penguin Life.

Fung, J. (2016). *The Obesity Code*. London, UK: Scribe.

Inchauspé, J. (2022). *Glucose Revolution*. London, UK: Short Books.

Jenkinson, A. (2021). *Why We Eat (Too Much)*. London, UK: Penguin Life.

Lustig, R. H. (2021). *Metabolical*. New York, NY: HarperWave.

Malhotra, A. (2021). *A Statin Free Life*. London, UK: Yellow Kite.

McMillan, J. (2017). *Get Lean, Stay Lean*. Sydney, Australia: Murdoch Books.

Nestor, J. (2020). *Breath*. London, UK: Penguin Life.

Panda, S. (2018). *The Circadian Code*. London, UK: Vermilion.

Saladino, D. (2021). *Eating to Extinction*. London, UK: Jonathan Cape.

Spector, T. D. (2020). *The Diet Myth*. London, UK: Weidenfeld & Nicolson.

Storoni, M. (2017). *Stress Proof*. New York, NY: TarcherPerigee.

ABOUT THE AUTHORS

Helen and Philip Bosanquet are siblings who work as doctors in the UK. Dr Helen Bosanquet graduated from Cardiff University School of Medicine in 2003. She worked in hospital medicine before moving into General Practice, qualifying in 2011. She holds a diploma in Lifestyle Medicine, and enjoys integrating lifestyle medicine into her current General Practice work. Dr Philip Bosanquet graduated from Southampton University School of Medicine in 2011, and qualified as a General Practitioner in 2016. Since then he has been working in both routine and urgent care GP settings, including for the 111 out-of-hours service.

Helen and Philip both live with their spouses and children in Lymington, on the south coast of England. They enjoy outdoor activity in their local area including walking in the New Forest National Park and swimming in the sea. They are both grateful to their parents, Andrew and Margie, who from a young age instilled in them a passion for healthy living, the natural world and family life.

Scan me for website

Printed in Great Britain
by Amazon

24905202R00064